UNRAVELING THE COOKBOOK SECRETS OF KETO AND LOW CARB LIVING

A GUIDE TO VIBRANT HEALTH

ANDRE RUTHERFORD

Unraveling the Cookbook Secrets of Keto and Low Carb Living

Copyright @2024 Andre Rutherford

All right reserved

Unraveling the Cookbook Secrets of Keto and Low Carb Living

Table Of Contents

CHAPTER ONE 1

INTRODUCTION TO KETO AND LOW CARB DIETS 1

    Origins of Keto and Low Carb Diets 1

    Principles of Keto and Low Carb Diets 1

    Scientific Rationale Behind Keto and Low Carb Diets 1

CHAPTER 2 1

GETTING STARTED WITH KETO AND LOW CARB DIETS 1

    Setting Goals and Expectations 1

    Kitchen Essentials for Keto and Low Carb Cooking 1

    Meal Planning and Prepping 1

CHAPTER 3 1

THE SCIENCE BEHIND KETO AND LOW CARB DIETS 1

    How Ketosis Works 1

    Macronutrient Ratios 1

Unraveling the Cookbook Secrets of Keto and Low Carb Living

Understanding Insulin and Blood Sugar 1

CHAPTER 4 1

FOODS TO EAT AND AVOID ON KETO AND LOW CARB DIETS 1

Keto-Friendly Foods 1

Healthy Fats 1

Protein Sources: 1

Low Carb Vegetables 1

Nuts and Seeds: 1

Dairy and Dairy Alternatives: 1

Low Carb Sweeteners: 1

Foods to Limit or Avoid 1

Refined Carbohydrates: 1

Sugary Beverages: 1

Processed Foods: 1

High Sugar Fruits: 1

Reading Labels and Making Smart Choices 1

CHAPTER 5 1

Unraveling the Cookbook Secrets of Keto and Low Carb Living

MEAL PLANS AND RECIPES FOR KETO AND LOW CARB DIETS 1

Sample Meal Plans for Beginners 1

Sample Meal Plan 1: 1

Day 1: 1

Day 2: 1

Sample Meal Plan 2: 1

Day 3: 1

Day 4 1

Quick and Easy Keto and Low Carb Recipes...1

Recipe 1: Keto Breakfast Casserole.............1

Recipe 2: Low Carb Chicken Alfred 1

CHAPTER 6 1

NAVIGATING SOCIAL SITUATIONS ON KETO AND LOW CARB DIETS..1

Eating Out on Keto..1

Keto-Friendly Travel Tips 1

Handling Social Events and Parties 1

CHAPTER 7 1

Unraveling the Cookbook Secrets of Keto and Low Carb Living

OVERCOMING CHALLENGES AND STAYING MOTIVATED ON KETO AND LOW CARB DIETS ...1

Dealing with Cravings and Temptations 1

Breaking Through Plateaus 1

Coping with Social Pressure and Judgment ...1

Staying Motivated for Long-Term Success......1

CHAPTER 8 1

ADVANCED STRATEGIES AND OPTIMIZATION TECHNIQUES FOR KETO AND LOW CARB DIETS.1

Tracking Macros and Nutrients......................1

Implementing Cyclical Ketogenic Diet (CKD) or Targeted Ketogenic Diet (TKD) 1

Practicing Intermittent Fasting (IF) 1

Experimenting with Supplemental Support...1

Practicing Mindful Eating and Stress Management 1

CHAPTER 9 1

TROUBLESHOOTING COMMON CHALLENGES AND PITFALLS ON KETO AND LOW CARB DIETS.1

Addressing Keto Flu and Transition Symptoms 1

Unraveling the Cookbook Secrets of Keto and Low Carb Living

Managing Digestive Issues and Gut Health....1

Overcoming Weight Loss Plateaus..................1

Finding Balance and Sustainability..................1

Navigating Social and Emotional Challenges .1

CHAPTER 10 1

PRACTICAL RESOURCES AND TOOLS FOR KETO AND LOW CARB SUCCESS 1

Meal Planning and Recipe Resources 1

Educational Websites and Online Courses 1

Tracking Tools and Apps 1

Supportive Communities and Social Networks 1

Additional Resources and Tools......................1

EMBRACING THE KETO AND LOW CARB LIFESTYLE FOR HEALTH AND WELLNESS 1

CHAPTER ONE

INTRODUCTION TO KETO AND LOW CARB DIETS

In recent years, the ketogenic (keto) and low carbohydrate (low carb) diets have gained immense popularity among individuals seeking to improve their health, lose weight, and enhance overall well-being. This chapter serves as an in-depth introduction to these dietary approaches, exploring their origins, principles, and the scientific rationale behind their effectiveness.

Origins of Keto and Low Carb Diets

The roots of the ketogenic diet can be traced back to the early 20th century when it was developed as a therapeutic intervention for epilepsy. In 1921, Dr. Russell Wilder, a physician at the Mayo Clinic, first introduced the concept of the ketogenic diet as a treatment for epilepsy patients who were not responding to conventional medications. By drastically reducing carbohydrate intake and increasing the consumption of fats, the ketogenic diet was found to induce a state of ketosis, which effectively reduced the frequency and severity of epileptic seizures in many patients.

Similarly, low carbohydrate diets have a long history, with variations emerging in different cultures and societies throughout the centuries. In the mid-19th century, William Banting, an English undertaker, popularized a low carbohydrate diet for weight loss, which he detailed in his pamphlet titled "Letter on Corpulence." Banting's diet, which emphasized the consumption of meat, fish, vegetables, and limited quantities of bread, sugar, and potatoes, foreshadowed the principles of modern low carb diets.

Principles of Keto and Low Carb Diets

At their core, both the ketogenic and low carb diets share a fundamental principle: the reduction of carbohydrate intake in favor of increased consumption of fats and proteins. By limiting carbohydrates, the body is forced to shift its primary fuel source from glucose to ketones, which are produced by the liver during the breakdown of fats.

The ketogenic diet typically consists of high-fat, moderate-protein, and very-low-carbohydrate foods. Carbohydrate intake is restricted to around 20-50 grams per day, primarily coming from non-starchy vegetables and small amounts of nuts and seeds. Fat intake is emphasized, with sources including avocados, nuts, seeds, olive oil, coconut oil, butter, and fatty cuts of meat.

Low carb diets, while also emphasizing reduced carbohydrate intake, may allow for slightly higher carbohydrate consumption compared to the ketogenic diet. However, the focus remains on minimizing the intake of refined carbohydrates, sugars, and processed foods, while prioritizing whole, nutrient-dense sources of carbohydrates such as vegetables, fruits, and legumes.

Scientific Rationale Behind Keto and Low Carb Diets

The effectiveness of keto and low carb diets can be attributed to their impact on metabolic processes within the body, particularly in relation to insulin, blood sugar levels, and fat metabolism.

When carbohydrates are consumed, they are broken down into glucose, which enters the bloodstream and stimulates the release of insulin from the pancreas. Insulin plays a crucial role in regulating blood sugar levels by facilitating the uptake of glucose into cells for energy production. However, chronically elevated insulin levels, often resulting from a diet high in carbohydrates, can lead to insulin resistance and metabolic dysfunction.

By reducing carbohydrate intake, particularly refined carbohydrates and sugars, keto and low carb diets help stabilize blood sugar levels and lower insulin secretion. This promotes fat burning and ketone production, leading to increased fat oxidation and weight loss. Additionally, ketones have been shown to have neuroprotective and anti-inflammatory effects, contributing to their therapeutic potential beyond weight management.

Furthermore, keto and low carb diets have been associated with numerous health benefits beyond weight loss, including improved blood lipid profiles, enhanced cognitive function, increased energy levels, and reduced risk factors for chronic diseases such as type 2 diabetes, cardiovascular disease, and metabolic syndrome.

In essence, keto and low carb diets represent powerful dietary strategies for achieving weight loss, optimizing health, and promoting overall wellness. By understanding their origins, principles, and underlying mechanisms, individuals can embark on a journey towards improved metabolic health and vitality through the adoption of these transformative dietary approaches.

CHAPTER 2

GETTING STARTED WITH KETO AND LOW CARB DIETS

Embarking on a ketogenic or low carbohydrate diet can be both exciting and daunting. This chapter is dedicated to providing readers with practical guidance on how to get started on their journey towards adopting and successfully implementing these dietary approaches. From setting clear goals and expectations to stocking the kitchen with essential ingredients, this chapter serves as a comprehensive roadmap for beginners.

Setting Goals and Expectations

Before diving into the world of keto and low carb diets, it's essential to establish clear goals and realistic expectations. Whether your primary objective is to lose weight, improve metabolic health, increase energy levels, or enhance overall well-being, defining your goals will help guide your dietary choices and measure progress along the way.

Begin by identifying specific, measurable, and achievable goals that align with your personal preferences and lifestyle. Consider factors such as desired weight loss targets, fitness goals, dietary preferences, and any underlying health conditions or concerns. By setting clear objectives, you'll be better equipped to stay motivated and focused on your journey towards success.

It's also important to manage expectations and understand that transitioning to a ketogenic or low carb diet may involve an adjustment period. While some individuals may experience rapid weight loss and immediate improvements in energy levels, others may require more time to adapt to the dietary changes and experience noticeable benefits. Be patient with yourself and trust the process, knowing that positive changes are unfolding within your body.

Kitchen Essentials for Keto and Low Carb Cooking

A well-equipped kitchen is essential for successfully navigating the world of keto and low carb cooking. Stocking up on the following essentials will ensure you have everything you need to prepare delicious and satisfying meals that adhere to your dietary goals:

Unraveling the Cookbook Secrets of Keto and
Low Carb Living

Healthy Fats: Incorporate a variety of healthy fats into your diet, including avocado oil, coconut oil, olive oil, grass-fed butter, ghee, and fatty cuts of meat. These fats will serve as the primary source of energy on a ketogenic diet and provide satiety and flavor to your meals.

Low Carb Vegetables: Fill your fridge with an assortment of low carb vegetables such as leafy greens, broccoli, cauliflower, zucchini, bell peppers, and asparagus. These nutrient-dense options are rich in fiber, vitamins, and minerals while being low in carbohydrates, making them ideal for keto and low carb diets.

Protein Sources: Choose high-quality protein sources to support muscle growth, repair, and satiety. Opt for pasture-raised eggs, grass-fed beef, wild-caught fish, poultry, tofu, tempeh, and legumes (in moderation for low carb diets).

Nuts and Seeds: Keep a selection of nuts and seeds on hand for snacking or adding crunch to salads and dishes. Almonds, walnuts, macadamia nuts, chia seeds, flaxseeds, and pumpkin seeds are excellent choices that provide healthy fats, protein, and fiber.

Low Carb Flours and Sweeteners: Experiment with alternative flours and sweeteners to create keto-friendly baked goods and desserts. Almond flour, coconut flour, and flaxseed meal can be used as substitutes for traditional wheat flour, while erythritol, stevia, and monk fruit sweeteners offer low glycemic options for satisfying your sweet tooth.

Herbs, Spices, and Condiments: Enhance the flavor of your meals with a variety of herbs, spices, and condiments. Stock up on staples such as garlic, ginger, turmeric, cumin, paprika, sea salt, black pepper, and sugar-free sauces and dressings to add depth and complexity to your dishes.

By ensuring your kitchen is well-stocked with these essential ingredients, you'll be prepared to tackle any recipe or meal with confidence and creativity.

Meal Planning and Prepping

Effective meal planning and prepping are key components of success on a ketogenic or low carbohydrate diet. By taking the time to plan your meals ahead of time and prepare ingredients in advance, you can save time, reduce stress, and stay on track with your dietary goals.

Start by creating a weekly meal plan that outlines breakfast, lunch, dinner, and snacks for each day of the week. Consider incorporating a

Unraveling the Cookbook Secrets of Keto and Low Carb Living

variety of proteins, healthy fats, and low carb vegetables into your meals to ensure balanced nutrition and satisfaction.

Once you have your meal plan in place, dedicate a specific day each week to grocery shopping and meal prepping. Take inventory of your pantry, fridge, and freezer, and make a list of any ingredients you need to purchase. Stick to the perimeter of the grocery store where you'll find fresh produce, meats, and dairy, and avoid the aisles filled with processed and high-carb foods.

When meal prepping, focus on batch-cooking proteins, chopping vegetables, and portioning out snacks and ingredients for easy grab-and-go meals throughout the week. Invest in quality storage containers to keep prepared meals fresh and organized, and label them with the date and contents for easy identification.

By adopting a proactive approach to meal planning and prepping, you'll streamline your cooking process, minimize food waste, and set yourself up for success on your keto or low carb journey.

Getting started with keto and low carb diets requires careful planning, preparation, and dedication. By setting clear goals and

Unraveling the Cookbook Secrets of Keto and Low Carb Living

expectations, stocking your kitchen with essential ingredients, and mastering the art of meal planning and prepping, you'll lay a solid foundation for achieving your desired health and wellness outcomes. Stay tuned for the following chapters, where we'll delve deeper into the science behind keto and low carb diets, explore the role of macronutrients, and provide practical tips for navigating social situations and overcoming challenges along the way.

CHAPTER 3

THE SCIENCE BEHIND KETO AND LOW CARB DIETS

Understanding the scientific principles that underpin keto and low carb diets is essential for maximizing their effectiveness and achieving desired health outcomes. In this chapter, we'll delve into the intricate mechanisms behind these dietary approaches, exploring how they impact metabolism, insulin sensitivity, and overall health.

How Ketosis Works

At the heart of the ketogenic diet lies the metabolic state known as ketosis. Ketosis occurs when the body shifts from primarily utilizing glucose as its primary fuel source to burning fat for energy. This metabolic adaptation is achieved through significant carbohydrate restriction, typically to less than 50 grams per day, which forces the body to rely on alternative fuel substrates, namely ketone bodies.

When carbohydrate intake is limited, glycogen stores in the liver are depleted, and insulin levels decrease. As a result, fatty acids are released from adipose tissue and transported to the liver, where they undergo a process called beta-oxidation to produce acetyl-CoA. Excess acetyl-CoA is then converted into ketone bodies, including acetoacetate, beta-hydroxybutyrate, and acetone, which are released into the bloodstream and used by tissues throughout the body as fuel.

Ketosis is characterized by elevated levels of circulating ketones, typically ranging from 0.5 to 3.0 mmol/L. This metabolic state offers several advantages, including increased fat oxidation, reduced reliance on glucose, and improved energy levels and mental clarity. Additionally, ketones have been shown to possess anti-inflammatory and neuroprotective properties, making ketosis a potentially therapeutic state for various health conditions.

Macronutrient Ratios

Central to the ketogenic and low carb diets is the manipulation of macronutrient ratios to promote ketosis and metabolic flexibility. While there is no one-size-fits-all approach to macronutrient distribution, typical ketogenic diets are characterized by high fat, moderate protein, and very low carbohydrate intake.

Unraveling the Cookbook Secrets of Keto and Low Carb Living

A standard ketogenic diet (SKD) typically consists of macronutrient ratios as follows:

- ★ Fat: 70-80% of total calories
- ★ Protein: 20-25% of total calories
- ★ Carbohydrate: 5-10% of total calories

In contrast, low carbohydrate diets may allow for slightly higher protein intake while still restricting carbohydrates. However, the emphasis remains on prioritizing healthy fats and minimizing carbohydrate consumption to induce and maintain ketosis.

It's important to note that individual macronutrient needs may vary based on factors such as age, gender, activity level, metabolic health, and weight loss goals. Experimentation and self-monitoring are key to finding the macronutrient ratios that work best for your unique physiology and preferences.

Understanding Insulin and Blood Sugar

Insulin plays a central role in regulating blood sugar levels and energy metabolism within the body. Produced by the pancreas in response to elevated blood glucose levels, insulin acts as a key that unlocks cells, allowing glucose to enter and be used for energy production or stored as glycogen or fat.

Unraveling the Cookbook Secrets of Keto and Low Carb Living

In individuals with insulin resistance or metabolic dysfunction, the body's cells become resistant to the effects of insulin, leading to chronically elevated blood sugar levels and increased insulin secretion. This dysregulation of insulin and blood sugar can contribute to weight gain, inflammation, and metabolic syndrome.

By reducing carbohydrate intake and minimizing spikes in blood sugar and insulin levels, keto and low carb diets help improve insulin sensitivity and promote metabolic health. By reducing the demand for insulin and stabilizing blood sugar levels, these dietary approaches can effectively manage and even reverse insulin resistance, leading to improved energy metabolism and reduced risk of chronic diseases such as type 2 diabetes and cardiovascular disease.

Furthermore, ketones have been shown to provide a more stable and sustained source of energy compared to glucose, leading to improved energy levels, mental clarity, and cognitive function. By promoting metabolic flexibility and reducing reliance on carbohydrates for fuel, keto and low carb diets offer a promising approach for optimizing health and well-being.

Unraveling the Cookbook Secrets of Keto and Low Carb Living

The science behind keto and low carb diets revolves around their ability to induce and maintain ketosis, manipulate macronutrient ratios to promote metabolic flexibility, and improve insulin sensitivity and blood sugar regulation. By understanding these underlying mechanisms, individuals can harness the power of these dietary approaches to achieve their desired health goals and unlock their full potential for vitality and wellness.

CHAPTER 4

FOODS TO EAT AND AVOID ON KETO AND LOW CARB DIETS

In Chapter 3, we explored the scientific principles behind keto and low carb diets. Now, let's dive into practical guidance on food choices, focusing on the types of foods to prioritize and those to limit or avoid to successfully adhere to these dietary approaches.

Keto-Friendly Foods

Adopting a ketogenic or low carb lifestyle doesn't mean sacrificing flavor or variety. In fact, there is a wide range of delicious and nutritious foods that are perfectly suited for these dietary approaches. Here are some keto-friendly foods to incorporate into your meal plan:

Healthy Fats

- Avocado: Rich in heart-healthy monounsaturated fats and fiber, avocados are a versatile ingredient that can be enjoyed in salads, smoothies, or as a spread.
- Olive Oil: A staple of Mediterranean cuisine, olive oil is an excellent source

of monounsaturated fats and antioxidants. Use it for cooking, salad dressings, or drizzling over roasted vegetables.
- Coconut Oil: Known for its medium-chain triglycerides (MCTs), coconut oil is a valuable addition to the keto diet. It can be used for cooking, baking, or adding flavor to smoothies and coffee.

Protein Sources:

Fatty Fish: Salmon, mackerel, sardines, and trout are rich in omega-3 fatty acids and high-quality protein. Aim to include fatty fish in your diet at least twice a week.

Grass-Fed Beef: Opt for grass-fed beef over conventionally raised varieties to maximize nutrient density and minimize exposure to antibiotics and hormones.

Poultry: Chicken, turkey, and duck are lean protein sources that can be enjoyed grilled, roasted, or sautéed with herbs and spices.

Low Carb Vegetables:

- ★ Leafy Greens: Spinach, kale, Swiss chard, and arugula are nutrient-dense options that are low in carbohydrates and high

in vitamins and minerals. Use them as a base for salads, stir-fries, or soups.
- ★ Cruciferous Vegetables: Broccoli, cauliflower, Brussels sprouts, and cabbage are rich in fiber and antioxidants. Roast them, steam them, or sauté them with garlic and olive oil for a tasty side dish.

Nuts and Seeds:

Almonds: Rich in healthy fats, protein, and fiber, almonds make a satisfying snack or crunchy topping for salads and yogurt.

Chia Seeds: Loaded with omega-3 fatty acids and soluble fiber, chia seeds are a nutritional powerhouse that can be added to smoothies, oatmeal, or baked goods.

Flaxseeds: High in lignans and alpha-linolenic acid (ALA), flaxseeds are beneficial for heart health and digestive function. Grind them and sprinkle them over yogurt or salads for a nutritional boost.

Dairy and Dairy Alternatives:

Full-Fat Yogurt: Choose plain, full-fat yogurt over flavored varieties to minimize added sugars. Greek yogurt is an excellent source of protein and probiotics.

Cheese: Enjoy a variety of cheeses, including cheddar, mozzarella, feta, and goat cheese, in moderation. Cheese adds flavor and richness to keto-friendly recipes.

Low Carb Sweeteners:

Stevia: A natural sweetener derived from the leaves of the Stevia rebaudiana plant, stevia is calorie-free and does not impact blood sugar levels.

Erythritol: A sugar alcohol that provides sweetness without the calories or glycemic effects of sugar, erythritol is commonly used in keto baking and desserts.

By incorporating these keto-friendly foods into your daily meals and snacks, you can enjoy a satisfying and varied diet while supporting your health and wellness goals.

Foods to Limit or Avoid

While there is a wide range of keto-friendly foods to choose from, there are also certain foods that are best limited or avoided altogether on keto and low carb diets. Here are some examples:

Refined Carbohydrates:

White Bread: High in refined carbohydrates and low in fiber, white bread can cause spikes in blood sugar levels and disrupt ketosis.

Pasta: Traditional pasta made from refined wheat flour is off-limits on keto and low carb diets due to its high carbohydrate content.

Sugary Snacks: Candy, cookies, cakes, and other sugary snacks are packed with empty calories and provide little nutritional value. They can also trigger cravings and sabotage weight loss efforts.

Sugary Beverages:

Soda: Regular soda is loaded with sugar and provides no nutritional benefits. Opt for sugar-free alternatives or sparkling water flavored with lemon or lime.

Fruit Juice: While natural fruit juice may seem healthy, it's often concentrated with sugar and lacks the fiber found in whole fruits. Choose water or herbal tea instead.

Starchy Vegetables:

Potatoes: Whether mashed, fried, or baked, potatoes are high in carbohydrates and can quickly derail ketosis. Substitute with lower carb options like cauliflower or turnips.

Corn: While technically a vegetable, corn is high in starch and sugar, making it unsuitable for keto and low carb diets.

Processed Foods:

Processed Meats: Hot dogs, deli meats, and other processed meats often contain added sugars, preservatives, and fillers that can hinder ketosis and contribute to inflammation.

Fast Food: Most fast food options are high in carbohydrates, unhealthy fats, and sodium. Opt for homemade meals prepared with whole, unprocessed ingredients whenever possible.

High Sugar Fruits:

Bananas: While bananas are a nutritious fruit, they are also high in carbohydrates and sugars. Enjoy them in moderation or choose lower carb fruits like berries or avocado.

Grapes: Grapes are another fruit that is relatively high in sugar and carbohydrates. Limit your intake or opt for smaller portions.

By being mindful of these foods to limit or avoid, you can maintain ketosis and stay on track with your dietary goals.

Reading Labels and Making Smart Choices

Unraveling the Cookbook Secrets of Keto and Low Carb Living

When following a ketogenic or low carb diet, it's essential to become proficient at reading food labels and identifying hidden sources of carbohydrates and sugars. Pay close attention to the following components:

- ★ Total Carbohydrates: Look for foods with low total carbohydrate counts, ideally less than 5-10 grams per serving. Be cautious of products labeled as "low carb" or "keto-friendly," as they may still contain hidden sugars and additives.
- ★ Fiber: Fiber is a type of carbohydrate that is not fully absorbed by the body and does not impact blood sugar levels. Aim to choose foods high in fiber to help promote feelings of fullness and support digestive health.
- ★ Sugar Alcohols: Sugar alcohols such as erythritol, xylitol, and sorbitol are commonly used as sweeteners in sugar-free and low carb products. While they provide sweetness without the calories or glycemic impact of sugar, they can cause digestive discomfort in some individuals when consumed in large amounts.
- ★ Artificial Sweeteners: Artificial sweeteners such as aspartame, sucralose, and saccharin are calorie-free

and do not impact blood sugar levels. While they are commonly used as sugar substitutes in diet sodas, sugar-free gum, and other processed foods, some research suggests that excessive consumption may have negative effects on metabolic health and gut microbiota. Exercise moderation when using artificial sweeteners and consider natural alternatives like stevia or monk fruit sweetener.

★ Serving Size: Pay attention to serving sizes listed on food labels, as they can vary significantly between products. Be mindful of portion sizes to avoid inadvertently consuming excess carbohydrates and sugars.

★ Ingredient List: Take a close look at the ingredient list to identify any hidden sources of carbohydrates, sugars, or additives. Choose foods with simple, whole-food ingredients and avoid products with lengthy lists of artificial preservatives, flavors, and colors.

By developing the habit of reading labels and making informed choices, you can navigate the grocery store aisles with confidence and ensure that you're selecting foods that align with your keto or low carb lifestyle.

Unraveling the Cookbook Secrets of Keto and Low Carb Living

Understanding which foods to prioritize and which to limit or avoid is essential for successfully adhering to a ketogenic or low carb diet. By incorporating nutrient-dense, whole foods rich in healthy fats, proteins, and low in carbohydrates, you can support your health and well-being while enjoying delicious and satisfying meals. By becoming proficient at reading labels and making smart choices, you can navigate the modern food landscape with confidence and empower yourself to achieve your dietary goals. Stay tuned for the following chapters, where we'll explore sample meal plans, recipes, and practical tips for meal prep and dining out on keto and low carb diets.

CHAPTER 5

MEAL PLANS AND RECIPES FOR KETO AND LOW CARB DIETS

Meal planning is a crucial component of success on keto and low carb diets. In this chapter, we'll provide sample meal plans and recipes to help you get started on your journey towards optimal health and wellness. From hearty breakfasts to satisfying dinners and everything in between, these meal ideas are designed to keep you nourished, satisfied, and on track with your dietary goals.

Sample Meal Plans for Beginners

Creating a well-balanced and varied meal plan is key to ensuring that you meet your nutritional needs while following a ketogenic or low carb diet. Here are two sample meal plans to help you kickstart your journey:

Sample Meal Plan 1:

Day 1:

- Breakfast: Scrambled eggs with spinach, mushrooms, and feta cheese cooked in olive oil.

- Lunch: Grilled chicken Caesar salad with romaine lettuce, cherry tomatoes, Parmesan cheese, and Caesar dressing.
- Dinner: Baked salmon with roasted asparagus and a side salad with mixed greens, avocado, and vinaigrette dressing.

Snack: Celery sticks with almond butter.

Day 2:

- Breakfast: Greek yogurt parfait with plain Greek yogurt, mixed berries, and a sprinkle of crushed almonds.
- Lunch: Turkey and avocado wrap using lettuce leaves as the wrap, filled with sliced turkey, avocado, tomato, and mayonnaise.
- Dinner: Zucchini noodles (zoodles) with marinara sauce and Italian sausage, topped with grated Parmesan cheese.
- Snack: Sliced cucumber with cream cheese and smoked salmon.

Sample Meal Plan 2:

Day 3:

- Breakfast: Keto-friendly smoothie made with coconut milk, spinach, avocado, protein powder, and chia seeds.

- Lunch: Taco salad with seasoned ground beef, shredded lettuce, diced tomatoes, shredded cheese, avocado slices, and salsa.
- Dinner: Baked chicken thighs with broccoli florets sautéed in garlic butter.
- Snack: Hard-boiled eggs with a sprinkle of salt and pepper.

Day 4:

- Breakfast: Crustless quiche made with eggs, bacon, spinach, and cheddar cheese.
- Lunch: Tuna salad lettuce wraps filled with canned tuna, diced celery, red onion, mayonnaise, and mustard.
- Dinner: Beef stir-fry with bell peppers, onions, broccoli, and cauliflower rice.
- Snack: Mixed nuts (almonds, walnuts, and pecans) with a piece of cheese.

Feel free to modify these meal plans based on your preferences, dietary restrictions, and nutritional needs. Experiment with different ingredients and flavor combinations to keep your meals exciting and enjoyable.

Unraveling the Cookbook Secrets of Keto and Low Carb Living

Quick and Easy Keto and Low Carb Recipes

In addition to sample meal plans, having a repertoire of quick and easy recipes is essential for maintaining variety and convenience in your keto or low carb lifestyle. Here are some delicious recipes to try:

Recipe 1: Keto Breakfast Casserole
Ingredients:

- 6 eggs
- 1/2 cup heavy cream
- 1 cup shredded cheddar cheese
- 1 cup cooked bacon or sausage, crumbled
- 1/2 cup diced bell peppers
- Salt and pepper to taste

Instructions:

Preheat your oven to 350°F (175°C). Grease a 9x9-inch baking dish.

In a large bowl, whisk together the eggs and heavy cream. Season with salt and pepper.

Stir in the shredded cheese, cooked bacon or sausage, and diced bell peppers.

Unraveling the Cookbook Secrets of Keto and Low Carb Living

Pour the mixture into the prepared baking dish and spread it out evenly.

Bake for 25-30 minutes, or until the casserole is set and golden brown on top.

Allow the casserole to cool slightly before slicing and serving. Enjoy hot or cold.

Recipe 2: Low Carb Chicken Alfredo

Ingredients:

- 4 boneless, skinless chicken breasts
- Salt and pepper to taste
- 2 tablespoons olive oil
- 2 cloves garlic, minced
- 1 cup heavy cream
- 1/2 cup grated Parmesan cheese
- 2 cups broccoli florets
- Fresh parsley for garnish

Instructions:

Season the chicken breasts with salt and pepper on both sides.

Heat the olive oil in a large skillet over medium heat. Add the chicken breasts and cook for 6-8 minutes per side, or until golden brown and cooked through. Remove from the skillet and set aside.

In the same skillet, add the minced garlic and sauté for 1-2 minutes, or until fragrant.

Pour in the heavy cream and bring to a simmer. Cook for 3-4 minutes, stirring occasionally, until the sauce has thickened slightly.

Stir in the grated Parmesan cheese until melted and smooth.

Add the broccoli florets to the skillet and cook for an additional 2-3 minutes, or until tender-crisp.

Return the cooked chicken breasts to the skillet and coat them in the Alfredo sauce.

Garnish with fresh parsley and serve hot.

Recipe 3: Keto Cauliflower Fried Rice

Ingredients:

- 1 head cauliflower, grated or finely chopped
- 2 tablespoons sesame oil
- 2 cloves garlic, minced
- 1 tablespoon grated ginger
- 2 cups mixed vegetables (such as bell peppers, carrots, and peas)

Unraveling the Cookbook Secrets of Keto and Low Carb Living

- 2 eggs, beaten
- 3 tablespoons soy sauce or tamari
- Salt and pepper to taste
- Sliced green onions for garnish

Instructions:

Heat the sesame oil in a large skillet or wok over medium heat. Add the minced garlic and grated ginger and sauté for 1-2 minutes, or until fragrant.

Add the mixed vegetables to the skillet and cook for 3-4 minutes, stirring occasionally, until tender.

Push the vegetables to one side of the skillet and add the beaten eggs to the empty side. Scramble the eggs until cooked through, then stir them into the vegetables.

Add the grated cauliflower to the skillet and stir to combine with the vegetables and eggs.

Pour the soy sauce or tamari over the cauliflower fried rice and stir to evenly coat.

Cook for an additional 5-6 minutes, stirring occasionally, until the cauliflower is tender and heated through.

Season with salt and pepper to taste, then garnish with sliced green onions before serving.

These recipes are just a starting point for your culinary adventures on keto and low carb diets. Feel free to customize them with your favorite ingredients and flavorings to suit your taste preferences.

By incorporating these sample meal plans and recipes into your weekly routine, you'll stay nourished, satisfied, and motivated on your journey towards optimal health and wellness. Experiment with different ingredients, flavors, and cooking techniques to keep your meals exciting and enjoyable, and don't be afraid to get creative in the kitchen. Stay tuned for the following chapters, where we'll explore practical tips for meal prep, dining out, and overcoming common challenges on keto and low carb diets.

CHAPTER 6

NAVIGATING SOCIAL SITUATIONS ON KETO AND LOW CARB DIETS

Following a ketogenic or low carb diet can present unique challenges, especially in social situations where food choices may be limited or tempting high-carb options are abundant. In this chapter, we'll explore practical strategies for navigating social gatherings, dining out, and traveling while staying true to your dietary goals. From communicating your needs to making informed choices, these tips will empower you to maintain your commitment to keto and low carb living in any social setting.

Eating Out on Keto

Dining out can be a delightful experience, but it often poses challenges for those following keto or low carb diets. Fortunately, with a little preparation and creativity, you can enjoy delicious meals at restaurants while staying within your dietary parameters.

Research Restaurants in Advance: Before heading out to eat, take some time to research restaurant menus online. Look for keto-friendly options such as grilled meats, seafood, salads, and vegetable sides. Many restaurants now offer low carb alternatives or are willing to accommodate special dietary requests.

Choose Wisely from the Menu: When dining out, focus on protein-rich dishes like grilled chicken, steak, or fish, paired with non-starchy vegetables or salads. Avoid dishes that are breaded, fried, or served with high-carb sauces or sides. Don't hesitate to ask your server about ingredient substitutions or modifications to fit your dietary needs.

Be Mindful of Hidden Carbs: While some dishes may seem keto-friendly at first glance, hidden sources of carbohydrates can sneak into restaurant meals through sauces, dressings, and garnishes. Ask for sauces and dressings on the side, or inquire about their ingredients to ensure they align with your dietary goals.

Practice Portion Control: Restaurant portions are often larger than what you would typically eat at home. Consider sharing an entrée with a dining companion or asking for a half portion to avoid overeating. You can also request a to-go box upfront and pack away half of your meal for later.

Unraveling the Cookbook Secrets of Keto and Low Carb Living

Stay Hydrated and Mindful: Drink plenty of water throughout your meal to stay hydrated and help curb cravings. Eat slowly and mindfully, savoring each bite and paying attention to hunger and fullness cues. Remember, it's okay to leave food on your plate if you're satisfied, even if others are still eating.

By employing these strategies, you can dine out with confidence while staying committed to your ketogenic or low carb lifestyle.

Keto-Friendly Travel Tips

Traveling presents additional challenges for maintaining a keto or low carb diet, but with careful planning and preparation, it's entirely possible to stay on track while exploring new destinations.

Pack Snacks and Portable Meals: Before embarking on your journey, pack a selection of keto-friendly snacks and portable meals to enjoy on the go. Options include nuts, seeds, beef jerky, cheese sticks, hard-boiled eggs, and pre-cut vegetables with dip. Having these snacks on hand will help you avoid the temptation of high-carb airport or gas station snacks.

Research Dining Options Ahead of Time: If possible, research restaurants and grocery stores at your destination that offer keto-friendly options. Look for salad bars, delis, and cafes that serve protein-rich salads, grilled meats, and vegetable sides. Many cities also have specialty grocery stores or health food stores where you can stock up on keto essentials.

Opt for Simple and Satisfying Meals: When dining out while traveling, opt for simple and satisfying meals that align with your dietary goals. Choose grilled meats, seafood, salads, and vegetable sides, and ask for modifications to accommodate your needs. Don't be afraid to communicate with restaurant staff about your dietary restrictions and preferences.

Stay Flexible and Adapt: While it's ideal to stick to your keto or low carb plan as much as possible, sometimes unexpected situations arise while traveling. Be flexible and adaptable, and don't stress too much if you're unable to find keto-friendly options for every meal. Focus on making the best choices available to you and enjoying the experience without guilt or restriction.

Plan Ahead for Special Occasions: If your travels coincide with special occasions or celebrations, plan ahead to ensure you can still enjoy the festivities while staying true to your dietary goals. Consider bringing keto-friendly snacks or treats to share with others, or offer to contribute a dish to the gathering that fits your dietary needs.

By following these travel tips and staying proactive in your planning, you can enjoy a seamless and stress-free keto or low carb experience while exploring new destinations.

Handling Social Events and Parties

Social events and parties are often centered around food and drinks, making them potential minefields for those following keto or low carb diets. However, with a little preparation and mindfulness, you can navigate these situations while still enjoying yourself.

Communicate Your Dietary Needs: If you're attending a social event where food will be served, consider reaching out to the host ahead of time to communicate your dietary needs. Offer to bring a keto-friendly dish to share or politely ask if they can accommodate your dietary preferences when planning the menu.

Focus on Socializing, Not Just Eating: While food may be a central focus of social gatherings, remember that the primary purpose is to connect and socialize with others. Shift your focus away from the food table and engage in meaningful conversations, games, or activities to distract yourself from temptation.

Have a Game Plan: Before attending a social event, have a game plan in place for how you'll navigate the food and drink options. Scan the menu or buffet table for keto-friendly options and prioritize those choices. Consider eating a small, protein-rich snack before arriving to help curb hunger and prevent overindulgence.

Choose Your Indulgences Wisely: It's okay to indulge in treats or alcoholic beverages occasionally, but choose your indulgences wisely and enjoy them mindfully. Opt for lower carb options like dry wine, spirits with zero-carb mixers, or keto-friendly desserts made with sugar substitutes. Be mindful of portion sizes and listen to your body's hunger and fullness cues.

Be Prepared to Navigate Peer Pressure and Judgment: In social settings, you may encounter peer pressure or judgment from others regarding your dietary choices. Remember that you're following a ketogenic or low carb diet for your health and well-being, and it's perfectly okay to prioritize your needs. Politely decline offers of high-carb foods or drinks, and confidently explain your dietary preferences if questioned. Educate others about the benefits of keto or low carb diets if they're genuinely interested, but don't feel obligated to justify or defend your choices to those who may not understand.

Stay Positive and Flexible: Finally, maintain a positive attitude and a flexible mindset when navigating social events and parties. Focus on the aspects of the gathering that bring you joy and connection, rather than fixating on food-related challenges or limitations. Remember that one meal or event does not define your overall progress or success on your keto or low carb journey. Stay committed to your goals, but also allow yourself to enjoy occasional indulgences and special occasions without guilt or self-judgment.

By applying these strategies and tips, you can confidently navigate social situations while staying true to your ketogenic or low carb lifestyle. With practice and experience, you'll develop the skills and resilience needed to thrive in any social setting, whether it's a family gathering, a night out with friends, or a festive holiday celebration. Embrace the opportunity to share your dietary journey with others and inspire them to prioritize their health and well-being as well.

CHAPTER 7

OVERCOMING CHALLENGES AND STAYING MOTIVATED ON KETO AND LOW CARB DIETS

Embarking on a ketogenic or low carb diet can be incredibly rewarding, but it's not without its challenges. From cravings and plateaus to social pressure and lifestyle adjustments, staying motivated and overcoming obstacles is essential for long-term success. In this chapter, we'll explore common challenges encountered on keto and low carb diets and provide practical strategies for staying motivated and resilient along the way.

Dealing with Cravings and Temptations

Cravings for high-carb foods are a common challenge faced by individuals on keto and low carb diets, especially during the initial transition period. Understanding the root causes of cravings and implementing strategies to manage them can help you stay on track with your dietary goals.

Identify Triggers: Pay attention to what triggers your cravings, whether it's stress, boredom, social situations, or specific food cues. Once you identify your triggers, you can develop alternative coping strategies to address them without turning to food.

Practice Mindful Eating: Slow down and pay attention to your hunger and fullness cues when eating. Mindful eating can help you savor your food more fully and prevent overeating or mindless snacking. Chew your food slowly, savoring each bite, and focus on the flavors and textures.

Choose Nutrient-Dense Foods: Prioritize nutrient-dense, whole foods that nourish your body and keep you satisfied for longer periods. Incorporate plenty of healthy fats, proteins, and fiber-rich vegetables into your meals to help stabilize blood sugar levels and reduce cravings.

Plan Ahead for Cravings: Anticipate cravings and have keto-friendly alternatives on hand to satisfy them. Keep a stash of low carb snacks like nuts, cheese, or dark chocolate for when cravings strike. Experiment with keto-friendly dessert recipes to indulge your sweet tooth without derailing your progress.

Stay Hydrated: Sometimes, feelings of hunger or cravings can be mistaken for thirst. Stay hydrated by drinking plenty of water throughout the day, and consider flavored sparkling water or herbal tea as a refreshing alternative.

By implementing these strategies, you can effectively manage cravings and stay committed to your ketogenic or low carb lifestyle.

Breaking Through Plateaus

Plateaus are a common occurrence on any weight loss journey, including keto and low carb diets. When you hit a plateau, it's essential to stay patient and persistent while implementing strategies to break through the stagnation.

Evaluate Your Progress: Take a step back and evaluate your dietary habits, activity levels, and overall lifestyle to identify areas for improvement. Are you accurately tracking your food intake? Are you getting enough exercise and sleep? Are there hidden sources of carbohydrates or sugars sneaking into your diet?

Adjust Your Macronutrient Ratios: If you've been following the same macronutrient ratios for an extended period without seeing results, consider adjusting your ratios slightly to kickstart progress. Experiment with increasing or decreasing your fat or protein intake while monitoring your body's response.

Incorporate Intermittent Fasting: Intermittent fasting, which involves cycling between periods of eating and fasting, can help break through weight loss plateaus by promoting fat burning and metabolic flexibility. Experiment with different fasting protocols, such as 16/8 or 24-hour fasts, to find what works best for you.

Increase Physical Activity: Amp up your exercise routine by incorporating more resistance training, cardiovascular exercise, or high-intensity interval training (HIIT) into your weekly regimen. Exercise not only burns calories but also helps build lean muscle mass and improve metabolic function.

Practice Stress Management: Chronic stress can contribute to weight loss plateaus by increasing cortisol levels and disrupting hormonal balance. Incorporate stress reducing activities such as meditation, yoga, deep breathing exercises, or spending time in nature to support your overall well-being.

By taking a proactive approach to breaking through plateaus and implementing targeted strategies, you can overcome stagnation and continue progressing towards your health and weight loss goals.

Coping with Social Pressure and Judgment

Navigating social situations while following a ketogenic or low carb diet can be challenging, especially when faced with pressure or judgment from others who may not understand or support your dietary choices. Here are some strategies for handling social pressure with confidence and resilience:

Educate and Communicate: Take the opportunity to educate others about the benefits of keto or low carb diets and explain why you've chosen to follow this lifestyle. Share your personal experiences, success stories, and the science behind these dietary approaches to dispel myths and misconceptions.

Set Boundaries: Be assertive in setting boundaries and advocating for your needs when faced with unsolicited advice or criticism. Politely decline offers of high-carb foods or drinks, and confidently assert your commitment to your dietary goals without feeling the need to justify or defend your choices.

Find Supportive Communities: Surround yourself with like-minded individuals who share your dietary values and can offer encouragement, motivation, and understanding.

Join online forums, social media groups, or local meetups dedicated to keto or low carb living to connect with others on similar journeys.

Lead by Example: Instead of succumbing to social pressure or judgment, lead by example and demonstrate the positive impact of your dietary choices through your actions and results. Focus on your own progress and well-being, and let your success speak for itself.

Practice Self-Compassion: Remember that your dietary journey is unique to you, and it's okay to make mistakes or deviate from your plan occasionally. Practice self-compassion and forgiveness, and don't be too hard on yourself if you encounter challenges along the way. Learn from setbacks and use them as opportunities for growth and self-improvement.

By implementing these strategies and staying true to your values and goals, you can confidently navigate social situations while staying committed to your ketogenic or low carb lifestyle.

Staying Motivated for Long-Term Success

Maintaining motivation and consistency over the long term is essential for achieving sustainable results on keto and low carb diets.

Here are some tips for staying motivated and committed to your dietary goals:

Set Clear and Realistic Goals: Establish clear, specific, and achievable goals that align with your values and priorities. Whether it's weight loss, improved health markers, increased energy levels, or better overall well-being, having a clear vision of what you want to achieve will help keep you motivated and focused.

Track Your Progress: Keep track of your progress over time by monitoring key metrics such as weight, body measurements, body fat percentage, and energy levels. Celebrate your successes, no matter how small, and use setbacks as learning opportunities to adjust your approach and keep moving forward.

Find Your Why: Identify your underlying reasons for wanting to follow a ketogenic or low carb diet and use them as motivation during challenging times. Whether it's improving your health, boosting your confidence, or setting a positive example for loved ones, connecting to your deeper purpose will help fuel your commitment and resilience.

Celebrate Non-Scale Victories: Don't solely rely on the scale to measure your progress.

Celebrate non-scale victories such as increased energy levels, improved sleep quality, better mood, enhanced mental clarity, and clothes fitting better as signs of progress and success.

Practice Self-Care: Prioritize self-care and nourish your body, mind, and soul with activities that bring you joy, relaxation, and fulfillment. Make time for hobbies, social connections, exercise, and other activities that contribute to your overall well-being and happiness. Taking care of yourself holistically will help you maintain a positive mindset and stay motivated to continue your keto or low carb journey.

Stay Educated and Informed: Stay informed about the latest research, trends, and developments in the field of ketogenic and low carb nutrition. Continuously educate yourself about the science behind these dietary approaches, as well as practical tips and strategies for success. Knowledge empowers you to make informed decisions and stay motivated on your journey.

Create a Supportive Environment: Surround yourself with supportive individuals who uplift and encourage you on your dietary journey. Whether it's family members, friends, or online communities, having a support network to lean on during challenging times can make a significant difference in your motivation and resilience.

Practice Resilience and Adaptability: Understand that setbacks and challenges are inevitable parts of any journey, including your dietary journey. Instead of viewing them as failures, see them as opportunities for growth and learning. Practice resilience and adaptability by bouncing back from setbacks quickly and adjusting your approach as needed.

Focus on Long-Term Health and Well-Being: Shift your focus from short-term results to long-term health and well-being. Instead of chasing rapid weight loss or quick fixes, prioritize sustainable lifestyle changes that support your overall health and longevity. Remember that true success is measured not just by the number on the scale, but by your overall quality of life.

Cultivate a Positive Mindset: Cultivate a positive mindset and believe in your ability to achieve your goals. Replace negative self-talk and limiting beliefs with affirmations, gratitude, and self-compassion. Visualize your success and stay optimistic about the possibilities that lie ahead.

Unraveling the Cookbook Secrets of Keto and Low Carb Living

By incorporating these strategies into your daily routine and mindset, you can stay motivated and resilient on your ketogenic or low carb journey for the long haul. Remember that your journey is unique to you, and progress may not always be linear. Stay committed, stay focused, and stay true to yourself as you work towards your health and wellness goals.

Overcoming challenges and staying motivated on ketogenic and low carb diets requires a combination of patience, perseverance, and mindset shifts. By implementing practical strategies for managing cravings, breaking through plateaus, handling social pressure, and staying motivated for long-term success, you can navigate your dietary journey with confidence and resilience. Embrace the journey, celebrate your progress, and trust in your ability to create lasting change in your life. Stay tuned for the following chapters, where we'll delve deeper into advanced strategies, troubleshooting tips, and practical resources for optimizing your ketogenic or low carb lifestyle.

CHAPTER 8

ADVANCED STRATEGIES AND OPTIMIZATION TECHNIQUES FOR KETO AND LOW CARB DIETS

As you progress on your ketogenic or low carb journey, you may find yourself seeking ways to optimize your results, overcome plateaus, and fine-tune your approach for maximum effectiveness. In this chapter, we'll explore advanced strategies and optimization techniques to help you take your keto or low carb lifestyle to the next level.

Tracking Macros and Nutrients

While initially focusing on keeping your carbohydrate intake low is crucial for entering and maintaining ketosis, as you become more experienced with the ketogenic or low carb diet, tracking your macronutrients (macros) and other key nutrients can provide valuable insights into your dietary habits and help you achieve your goals more effectively.

Calculate Your Macros: Determine your personalized macronutrient ratios based on your goals, activity level, age, gender, and metabolic needs. The standard ketogenic diet typically consists of around 70-75% of calories from fat, 20-25% from protein, and 5-10% from carbohydrates. Experiment with different ratios to find what works best for you.

Use Tracking Tools: Utilize tracking apps or websites to log your daily food intake and track your macros and nutrient intake. These tools can help you stay accountable, identify potential deficiencies or imbalances, and make informed adjustments to your diet as needed.

Focus on Quality and Variety: While tracking macros is essential, don't overlook the importance of nutrient quality and variety in your diet. Aim to consume a wide range of whole, nutrient-dense foods such as leafy greens, non-starchy vegetables, lean proteins, healthy fats, and low glycemic index fruits. Prioritize quality over quantity when it comes to food choices.

Monitor Electrolytes: Electrolyte imbalances, particularly sodium, potassium, and magnesium, are common on ketogenic diets due to increased fluid loss and reduced insulin levels. Monitor your electrolyte intake and consider supplementing with electrolyte-rich foods or supplements if necessary to prevent symptoms like fatigue, muscle cramps, or headaches.

Adjust as Needed: Pay attention to your body's response to different macronutrient ratios and adjust your intake accordingly. If you're experiencing stalls in weight loss or other symptoms, experiment with tweaking your fat, protein, or carbohydrate intake to find the optimal balance for your individual needs.

By tracking your macros and nutrients, you can gain valuable insights into your dietary habits, optimize your nutrient intake, and fine-tune your approach for maximum effectiveness on your ketogenic or low carb journey.

Implementing Cyclical Ketogenic Diet (CKD) or Targeted Ketogenic Diet (TKD)

While the standard ketogenic diet (SKD) involves consistently maintaining a low-carb, high-fat diet to achieve and sustain ketosis, some individuals may benefit from incorporating variations such as the cyclical ketogenic diet (CKD) or targeted ketogenic diet (TKD) for specific purposes, such as athletic performance, muscle building, or metabolic flexibility.

Cyclical Ketogenic Diet (CKD): CKD involves cycling between periods of strict ketogenic eating and higher-carb refeed days. Typically, individuals follow a standard ketogenic diet for 5-6 days of the week, followed by 1-2 days of higher carbohydrate intake. This cyclical approach allows for glycogen replenishment, supports intense workouts, and may help prevent metabolic adaptation to long-term ketosis.

Targeted Ketogenic Diet (TKD): TKD involves consuming a small amount of carbohydrates around workouts to provide a quick source of energy for performance without disrupting ketosis. Typically, individuals consume 15-30 grams of fast-digesting carbohydrates, such as glucose or dextrose, before or after intense exercise sessions. This targeted approach can enhance workout performance and recovery while still maintaining ketosis during the rest of the day.

Assess Your Goals and Needs: Before implementing CKD or TKD, carefully assess your goals, activity level, and individual needs. CKD may be more suitable for individuals engaged in high-intensity exercise or sports that require glycogen stores for performance, while TKD may be beneficial for those looking to optimize workout performance without sacrificing ketosis.

Experiment and Monitor: If considering CKD or TKD, experiment with different protocols and monitor your body's response closely. Pay attention to changes in energy levels, performance, body composition, and ketone levels to determine the effectiveness of these strategies for your goals.

Consult with a Professional: Before making significant changes to your dietary approach, especially if you have underlying health conditions or specific goals, consult with a qualified healthcare professional or registered dietitian who can provide personalized guidance and support.

By implementing variations such as CKD or TKD strategically and in alignment with your goals and needs, you can potentially enhance performance, muscle growth, and metabolic flexibility while still reaping the benefits of ketogenic or low carb living.

Practicing Intermittent Fasting (IF)

Intermittent fasting (IF) is a dietary approach that involves cycling between periods of eating and fasting, with various fasting and feeding windows. When combined with a ketogenic or low carb diet, intermittent fasting can further enhance fat burning, improve metabolic health, and promote overall well-being.

Choose Your Fasting Protocol: There are several different intermittent fasting protocols to choose from, including the 16/8 method (16 hours of fasting, 8-hour eating window), the 24-hour fast (fasting for a full day), alternate-day fasting (alternating between fasting and eating days), and more. Experiment with different protocols to find what works best for your schedule and preferences.

Start Slowly and Gradually: If new to intermittent fasting, start with shorter fasting periods and gradually increase the duration as your body adapts. Begin with a 12-hour overnight fast and gradually extend it to 14, 16, or more hours over time. Listen to your body's hunger and fullness cues and adjust your fasting window accordingly.

Stay Hydrated: During fasting periods, stay hydrated by drinking plenty of water, herbal tea, or black coffee. Hydration is essential for supporting metabolic function, energy levels, and overall well-being during fasting.

Focus on Nutrient-Dense Meals: When breaking your fast, prioritize nutrient-dense, whole foods that provide essential vitamins, minerals, and macronutrients. Incorporate plenty of healthy fats, lean proteins, non-starchy vegetables, and low glycemic index carbohydrates to support satiety, energy levels, and overall health.

Monitor Your Body's Response: Pay attention to how your body responds to intermittent fasting, including changes in energy levels, hunger cues, mood, and cognitive function. If you experience any negative symptoms or discomfort, consider adjusting your fasting protocol or consulting with a healthcare professional.

By incorporating intermittent fasting strategically into your ketogenic or low carb lifestyle, you can amplify the benefits of both approaches and optimize your metabolic health, weight loss, and overall well-being.

Experimenting with Supplemental Support

While a well-formulated ketogenic or low carb diet provides the majority of essential nutrients your body needs for optimal health, certain supplements may offer additional support, especially for addressing specific needs or deficiencies. Here are some key supplements to consider incorporating into your routine:

Electrolytes: As mentioned earlier, electrolyte imbalances are common on ketogenic diets due to increased fluid loss and reduced insulin levels. Consider supplementing with electrolytes such as sodium, potassium, and magnesium to support hydration balance and prevent symptoms like fatigue, muscle cramps, or headaches. Look for electrolyte supplements specifically formulated for ketogenic or low carb dieters, or incorporate electrolyte-rich foods such as leafy greens, nuts, seeds, and avocados into your diet.

Omega-3 Fatty Acids: Omega-3 fatty acids, found in fatty fish like salmon, mackerel, and sardines, as well as fish oil supplements, are essential for supporting heart health, brain function, and inflammation management. Consider supplementing with high-quality fish oil or algae oil to ensure adequate intake of these beneficial fats.

Vitamin D: Many individuals, especially those living in northern latitudes or spending limited time outdoors, may be deficient in vitamin D, which is essential for bone health, immune function, and mood regulation. Consider supplementing with vitamin D3, particularly during the winter months, or spend time outdoors to naturally increase your vitamin D levels.

B Vitamins: B vitamins play a crucial role in energy production, metabolism, and nerve function. While a well-rounded ketogenic or low carb diet typically provides ample B vitamins from foods like meat, fish, eggs, and leafy greens, supplementing with a B-complex vitamin or individual B vitamins such as B12 or folate may be beneficial, especially for vegetarians or individuals with absorption issues.

Probiotics: Gut health is essential for overall well-being, and maintaining a healthy balance of gut bacteria is crucial for digestion, immune function, and inflammation regulation. Consider supplementing with a high-quality probiotic to support gut health, particularly if you've experienced digestive issues or have recently taken antibiotics.

Adaptogens: Adaptogens are herbal compounds that help the body adapt to stress and promote balance and resilience. Popular adaptogens include ashwagandha, rhodiola, and holy basil, which may help support energy levels, reduce stress, and improve mental clarity. Incorporate adaptogenic herbs into your routine through supplements or herbal teas to support your body's stress response.

Consult with a Healthcare Professional: Before incorporating any new supplements into your routine, especially if you have underlying health conditions or are taking medications, consult with a qualified healthcare professional or registered dietitian. They can provide personalized recommendations based on your individual needs, goals, and health status.

By strategically incorporating supplements into your ketogenic or low carb lifestyle, you can address specific needs, optimize your nutrient intake, and support your overall health and well-being.

Practicing Mindful Eating and Stress Management

In addition to focusing on macronutrients, supplements, and dietary strategies, practicing mindful eating and stress management techniques can further enhance your ketogenic or low carb journey by promoting overall well-being and optimizing metabolic function.

Mindful Eating: Mindful eating involves paying attention to your food choices, hunger cues, and eating habits without judgment or distraction. Practice mindful eating by slowing down, savoring each bite, and paying attention to hunger and fullness cues. Avoid distractions like screens or multitasking while eating, and tune into the sensory experience of eating.

Stress Management: Chronic stress can negatively impact metabolism, hormone balance, and appetite regulation, making it more challenging to achieve and maintain ketosis. Incorporate stress management techniques such as meditation, deep breathing exercises, yoga, or journaling into your daily routine to promote relaxation and resilience.

Prioritize Sleep: Quality sleep is essential for overall health and metabolic function, including hormone regulation, appetite control, and energy levels. Aim for 7-9 hours of restful sleep per night, and establish a consistent sleep schedule and bedtime routine to support optimal sleep quality and duration.

Practice Gratitude and Self-Compassion: Cultivate a mindset of gratitude and self-compassion as you navigate your ketogenic or low carb journey. Focus on the positive aspects of your progress and celebrate your successes, no matter how small. Practice self-care and kindness towards yourself, and forgive yourself for any setbacks or challenges along the way.

Seek Support and Connection: Surround yourself with supportive individuals who uplift and encourage you on your dietary journey. Share your experiences, challenges, and successes with friends, family members, or online communities who understand and support your goals. Seek professional support from a therapist or counselor if you're struggling with emotional eating or stress-related issues.

By prioritizing mindful eating, stress management, and self-care practices, you can support your overall well-being and optimize your ketogenic or low carb lifestyle for long-term success and sustainability.

Implementing advanced strategies and optimization techniques such as tracking macros and nutrients, incorporating variations like cyclical ketogenic diet (CKD) or targeted ketogenic diet (TKD), experimenting with intermittent fasting (IF), supplementing strategically, and practicing mindful eating and stress management can help you take your ketogenic or low carb journey to the next level.

Unraveling the Cookbook Secrets of Keto and Low Carb Living

By combining these approaches with a personalized, holistic approach to health and wellness, you can achieve lasting results and thrive on your dietary journey for years to come. Stay tuned for the following chapters, where we'll delve deeper into troubleshooting tips, practical resources, and additional strategies for optimizing your ketogenic or low carb lifestyle.

CHAPTER 9

TROUBLESHOOTING COMMON CHALLENGES AND PITFALLS ON KETO AND LOW CARB DIETS

While the ketogenic and low carb diets offer numerous benefits, they can also present challenges and pitfalls that may hinder progress and success. In this chapter, we'll explore common issues faced by individuals following keto and low carb diets and provide practical solutions and troubleshooting tips to help you overcome obstacles and stay on track towards your health and wellness goals.

Addressing Keto Flu and Transition Symptoms

One of the most common challenges encountered when starting a ketogenic diet is the onset of symptoms often referred to as "keto flu." These symptoms can include fatigue, headache, dizziness, nausea, irritability, and brain fog, and typically occur during the initial transition period as your body adjusts to using ketones for fuel instead of glucose.

Stay Hydrated and Electrolyte Balanced: Dehydration and electrolyte imbalances are common contributors to keto flu symptoms. Increase your water intake and ensure adequate electrolyte intake by consuming foods rich in sodium, potassium, and magnesium, or by supplementing with electrolyte powders or tablets.

Gradually Reduce Carbohydrates: Instead of drastically cutting carbohydrates overnight, gradually reduce your carb intake over a period of days or weeks to allow your body to adapt more smoothly. Start by reducing high-carb foods like bread, pasta, and sugar, and gradually increase your intake of healthy fats and proteins.

Increase Healthy Fat Intake: Incorporate plenty of healthy fats into your meals to provide sustained energy and support ketone production. Include sources of healthy fats such as avocados, olive oil, coconut oil, nuts, seeds, and fatty fish in your diet to promote satiety and reduce cravings.

Get Sufficient Rest and Sleep: Prioritize rest and quality sleep during the initial transition period to support your body's adaptation to ketosis. Aim for 7-9 hours of sleep per night and establish a consistent sleep schedule to promote optimal rest and recovery.

Be Patient and Persistent: Understand that keto flu symptoms are temporary and typically subside within a few days to a week as your body adjusts to using ketones for fuel. Be patient with yourself during this transition period and focus on nourishing your body with nutrient-dense foods to support overall well-being.

By implementing these strategies and supporting your body's transition to ketosis, you can minimize keto flu symptoms and ease the transition into your ketogenic lifestyle.

Managing Digestive Issues and Gut Health

Some individuals may experience digestive issues such as constipation, diarrhea, bloating, or gas when starting a ketogenic or low carb diet. These issues can be attributed to various factors, including changes in dietary fiber intake, altered gut microbiota, or insufficient hydration.

Increase Fiber-Rich Foods: Focus on incorporating plenty of fiber-rich, non-starchy vegetables into your meals to support digestive health and regularity.

Include vegetables such as leafy greens, broccoli, cauliflower, Brussels sprouts, and asparagus, which provide essential nutrients and promote healthy digestion.

Stay Hydrated: Adequate hydration is essential for maintaining healthy digestion and preventing constipation. Drink plenty of water throughout the day, and consider incorporating hydrating foods like cucumbers, celery, and watermelon into your diet to support hydration and gut health.

Consider Probiotic Foods: Probiotic-rich foods such as yogurt, kefir, sauerkraut, kimchi, and kombucha contain beneficial bacteria that support gut health and digestion. Consider incorporating these foods into your diet regularly to promote a healthy balance of gut microbiota.

Monitor Fat Intake: While healthy fats are a staple of ketogenic diets, excessive fat intake, particularly from sources like dairy or MCT oil, can sometimes contribute to digestive issues or discomfort. Monitor your fat intake and experiment with adjusting the types and amounts of fats in your diet to find what works best for your digestion.

Practice Mindful Eating: Slow down and chew your food thoroughly, allowing your body time to digest and assimilate nutrients properly. Avoid overeating or consuming large meals too quickly, as this can put strain on your digestive system and exacerbate digestive issues.

By prioritizing fiber-rich foods, staying hydrated, incorporating probiotic-rich foods, monitoring fat intake, and practicing mindful eating habits, you can support digestive health and minimize discomfort while following a ketogenic or low carb diet.

Overcoming Weight Loss Plateaus

Weight loss plateaus are common on any dietary regimen, including ketogenic and low carb diets, and can be frustrating for individuals striving to reach their weight loss goals. However, plateaus are often temporary and can be overcome with strategic adjustments to your diet and lifestyle.

Reassess Your Macros: If you've hit a weight loss plateau, reassess your macronutrient intake and adjust your ratios as needed. Consider slightly reducing your fat intake or increasing your protein intake to promote fat burning and support muscle preservation.

Practice Intermittent Fasting: Incorporating intermittent fasting into your routine can help break through weight loss plateaus by promoting fat burning and metabolic flexibility. Experiment with different fasting protocols, such as 16/8 or 24-hour fasts, to find what works best for your body.

Increase Physical Activity: Amp up your exercise routine by incorporating more resistance training, cardiovascular exercise, or high-intensity interval training (HIIT) into your weekly regimen. Exercise not only burns calories but also helps build lean muscle mass and improve metabolic function.

Evaluate Your Caloric Intake: While ketogenic and low carb diets typically promote satiety and spontaneous calorie reduction, it's still possible to overconsume calories, especially if relying heavily on high-fat, calorie-dense foods. Track your food intake and reassess your portion sizes to ensure you're in a calorie deficit for weight loss.

Manage Stress and Sleep: Chronic stress and inadequate sleep can contribute to weight loss plateaus by disrupting hormone balance and metabolism. Prioritize stress management techniques such as meditation, yoga, or deep breathing exercises, and aim for 7-9 hours of quality sleep per night to support optimal metabolic function and weight loss.

By implementing these strategies and making targeted adjustments to your diet and lifestyle, you can overcome weight loss plateaus and continue progressing towards your health and wellness goals on your ketogenic or low carb journey.

Finding Balance and Sustainability

Maintaining balance and sustainability is key to long-term success on ketogenic and low carb diets. While these dietary approaches offer numerous benefits, it's essential to find a balance that works for your individual needs, preferences, and lifestyle to ensure lasting results and overall well-being.

Focus on Whole, Nutrient-Dense Foods: Prioritize whole, nutrient-dense foods such as lean proteins, healthy fats, non-starchy vegetables, and low glycemic index fruits to provide essential nutrients and promote overall health. While keto-friendly processed foods and snacks can be convenient occasionally, aim to primarily nourish your body with real, whole foods.

Allow for Flexibility and Variety: While consistency is crucial for success on ketogenic and low carb diets, allowing for flexibility and variety in your meal choices can prevent feelings of deprivation and promote long-term adherence. Experiment with different recipes, cuisines, and meal plans to keep your meals interesting and enjoyable.

Practice Mindful Eating and Intuitive Eating: Listen to your body's hunger and fullness cues and practice mindful eating to promote a healthy relationship with food. Avoid restrictive dieting behaviors or rigid meal plans, and instead focus on nourishing your body with balanced, satisfying meals that support your health and well-being. Trust your body's innate wisdom and intuition when making food choices, and prioritize pleasure and satisfaction in your eating experience.

Incorporate Social and Cultural Factors: Recognize that social gatherings, holidays, and cultural traditions may present challenges or temptations when following a ketogenic or low carb diet. Instead of viewing these occasions as obstacles, find ways to adapt and participate while staying true to your dietary goals. Bring keto-friendly dishes to potlucks or family gatherings, or communicate your dietary preferences and needs with hosts in advance.

Embrace a Holistic Approach to Health: Remember that health is about more than just what you eat. Prioritize other aspects of health and well-being, such as stress management, sleep quality, physical activity, social connections, and mental and emotional well-being. Cultivate a holistic approach to health that integrates all aspects of wellness for optimal vitality and longevity.

Seek Professional Guidance and Support: If you're struggling to find balance or sustainability on your ketogenic or low carb journey, don't hesitate to seek professional guidance and support. Consult with a registered dietitian, nutritionist, or healthcare provider who specializes in ketogenic or low carb nutrition to receive personalized recommendations and guidance tailored to your individual needs and goals.

By finding balance, flexibility, and sustainability in your approach to ketogenic or low carb living, you can achieve long-term success and enjoy the many benefits of these dietary lifestyles without feeling deprived or restricted.

Navigating Social and Emotional Challenges

Social and emotional challenges can arise when following a ketogenic or low carb diet, particularly in social settings or during times of stress or emotional upheaval. Learning to navigate these challenges with resilience and grace is essential for maintaining consistency and adherence to your dietary goals.

Communicate Your Needs: Be open and honest with friends, family members, and loved ones about your dietary preferences and needs. Educate them about the benefits of ketogenic or low carb diets and communicate how they can support you in your journey. Express your gratitude for their understanding and willingness to accommodate your dietary choices.

Plan Ahead for Social Gatherings: Before attending social events or gatherings, plan ahead by researching the menu or offering to bring a keto-friendly dish to share. By proactively preparing for social situations, you can ensure that you have options available that align with your dietary goals and preferences.

Practice Mindful Eating: Practice mindfulness and self-awareness when navigating social situations involving food. Be mindful of your hunger and fullness cues, and choose foods that nourish your body and align with your dietary goals. Focus on enjoying the company of others rather than fixating on food-related challenges.

Develop Coping Strategies: Develop coping strategies for dealing with social pressure, cravings, or emotional eating triggers. Find alternative ways to cope with stress or emotions, such as practicing deep breathing exercises, going for a walk, journaling, or calling a supportive friend.

Practice Self-Compassion: Be kind to yourself and practice self-compassion when faced with challenges or setbacks on your dietary journey. Remember that perfection is not attainable, and it's okay to make mistakes or deviate from your plan occasionally. Treat yourself with the same kindness and understanding that you would offer to a friend.

By developing effective communication skills, planning ahead for social gatherings, practicing mindful eating, developing coping strategies, and practicing self-compassion, you can navigate social and emotional challenges with confidence and resilience while staying true to your ketogenic or low carb lifestyle.

Troubleshooting common challenges and pitfalls on ketogenic and low carb diets requires a combination of practical strategies, mindset shifts, and self-awareness. By addressing issues such as keto flu symptoms, digestive issues, weight loss plateaus, finding balance and sustainability, and navigating social and emotional challenges with resilience and grace, you can overcome obstacles and stay on track towards your health and wellness goals. Embrace the journey, celebrate your progress, and trust in your ability to overcome challenges and thrive on your ketogenic or low carb journey. Stay tuned for the following chapters, where we'll delve deeper into practical resources, advanced strategies, and additional tips for optimizing your ketogenic or low carb lifestyle.

CHAPTER 10

PRACTICAL RESOURCES AND TOOLS FOR KETO AND LOW CARB SUCCESS

In this chapter, we'll explore a variety of practical resources and tools to support your success on the ketogenic or low carb diet. From meal planning apps to educational websites, these resources can provide valuable information, guidance, and support as you navigate your dietary journey.

Meal Planning and Recipe Resources

Meal planning is essential for success on any dietary regimen, including ketogenic and low carb diets. Having a variety of delicious and nutritious recipes at your fingertips can make meal prep easier and more enjoyable. Here are some valuable resources for meal planning and recipe inspiration:

Keto and Low Carb Recipe Websites: Explore websites dedicated to ketogenic and low carb recipes, such as Diet Doctor, ruled.me, and Wholesome Yum. These websites offer a wide range of recipes, from breakfasts and snacks to main courses and desserts, all tailored to fit within keto or low carb parameters.

Recipe Books and Cookbooks: Invest in recipe books or cookbooks focused on ketogenic or low carb cooking. Look for titles by reputable authors and chefs who specialize in these dietary approaches, and choose books that feature simple, flavorful recipes with easy-to-find ingredients.

Meal Planning Apps: Utilize meal planning apps such as Carb Manager, MyFitnessPal, or Cronometer to track your macros, plan your meals, and discover new recipes. These apps often provide features like barcode scanning, recipe importing, and meal logging to streamline the meal planning process.

Social Media and Online Communities: Join social media groups and online communities dedicated to ketogenic or low carb living, where members share recipes, meal ideas, tips, and success stories. Platforms like Instagram, Facebook, and Reddit are excellent places to connect with like-minded individuals and find inspiration for your meals.

Cooking Shows and YouTube Channels: Watch cooking shows or YouTube channels focused on ketogenic or low carb cooking for recipe inspiration and culinary tips. Many chefs and content creators share step-by-step tutorials and meal prep ideas that cater to specific dietary preferences and restrictions.

By leveraging these meal planning and recipe resources, you can streamline your meal prep process, discover new culinary creations, and stay inspired and motivated on your ketogenic or low carb journey.

Educational Websites and Online Courses

Educating yourself about the science behind ketogenic and low carb diets, as well as practical tips and strategies for success, is essential for making informed decisions and staying motivated on your dietary journey. Here are some valuable educational resources to explore:

- Ketogenic and Low Carb Websites: Dive into educational websites dedicated to ketogenic and low carb nutrition, such as The Ketogenic Diet Resource, KetoConnect, or KetoDiet Blog. These websites offer a wealth of information on the science behind ketosis, meal planning, troubleshooting common issues, and more.

- Online Courses and Webinars: Enroll in online courses or webinars focused on ketogenic or low carb nutrition, led by experts in the field. Look for courses that cover topics such as the fundamentals of ketosis, meal planning strategies, cooking techniques, and practical tips for success.
- Scientific Journals and Research Articles: Explore scientific journals and research articles to deepen your understanding of the physiological effects of ketogenic and low carb diets. Websites like PubMed or Google Scholar allow you to search for peer-reviewed studies on topics such as metabolic health, weight loss, and disease prevention.
- Podcasts and Audio Resources: Listen to podcasts or audio resources dedicated to ketogenic or low carb living for on-the-go education and inspiration. Many podcasts feature interviews with leading experts, success stories from individuals following these dietary approaches, and practical tips for implementation.
- Online Forums and Discussion Boards: Engage with online forums and discussion boards where individuals

share their experiences, ask questions, and provide support related to ketogenic or low carb diets. Websites like Reddit's r/keto or forums on keto-focused websites offer valuable insights and community camaraderie.

By immersing yourself in educational resources and staying informed about the latest research and developments in ketogenic and low carb nutrition, you can empower yourself to make informed decisions and optimize your dietary approach for success.

Tracking Tools and Apps

Tracking your food intake, macros, and progress can provide valuable insights into your dietary habits and help you stay accountable and motivated on your ketogenic or low carb journey. Here are some useful tracking tools and apps to consider:

- ★ Macronutrient Tracking Apps: Use apps such as MyFitnessPal, Carb Manager, or Cronometer to track your daily food intake and monitor your macronutrient ratios. These apps allow you to set personalized goals, log your meals, and track your progress towards achieving ketosis or low carb targets.

- ★ Ketone and Glucose Monitoring Devices: Invest in ketone and glucose monitoring devices such as blood ketone meters or breath ketone analyzers to track your ketone levels and ensure you're in a state of ketosis. These devices provide real-time feedback on your metabolic status and can help you optimize your dietary approach.
- ★ Fitness Trackers and Wearable Devices: Use fitness trackers or wearable devices to monitor your physical activity, sleep patterns, and overall health metrics. Many fitness trackers offer features like step counting, heart rate monitoring, and sleep tracking to help you stay active and prioritize recovery.
- ★ Food Diary and Journaling Apps: Keep a food diary or journal using apps like Evernote, MyPlate, or Lose It! to track your meals, snacks, cravings, and emotions. Journaling can help you identify patterns, triggers, and areas for improvement in your dietary habits and mindset.
- ★ Progress Photo Apps: Take progress photos regularly using apps like Progress, BodyShot, or Transformation to visually track your body composition changes over time. Progress photos can

serve as a powerful motivator and reminder of how far you've come on your ketogenic or low carb journey.
- ★ By incorporating tracking tools and apps into your routine, you can gain valuable insights into your dietary habits, monitor your progress towards your goals, and stay accountable and motivated on your ketogenic or low carb journey.

Supportive Communities and Social Networks

Finding support and camaraderie from like-minded individuals can make a significant difference in your success and adherence to ketogenic or low carb diets. Joining supportive communities and social networks allows you to connect with others, share experiences, ask questions, and find encouragement and inspiration along the way. Here are some ways to tap into supportive communities:

- Social Media Groups: Join Facebook groups, Instagram communities, or Twitter chats dedicated to ketogenic or low carb living. These groups provide a platform for connecting with others,

sharing recipes and tips, and receiving support and encouragement from fellow members.
- Online Forums and Discussion Boards: Engage with online forums and discussion boards focused on ketogenic or low carb diets, such as Reddit's r/keto or forums on keto-friendly websites. These platforms allow you to ask questions, share experiences, and connect with a diverse community of individuals following similar dietary approaches.
- Local Meetup Groups: Seek out local meetup groups or gatherings for individuals interested in ketogenic or low carb lifestyles. Meetup.com or social media platforms often feature groups organized by geographic location, where members can meet in person for support, camaraderie, and shared activities.
- Workshops and Events: Attend workshops, seminars, or events dedicated to ketogenic or low carb nutrition, where you can learn from experts, connect with peers, and participate in hands-on activities. Look for events hosted by reputable

- Accountability Partners or Buddy Systems: Pair up with an accountability partner or buddy system who shares similar goals and dietary preferences. Accountability partners can provide support, motivation, and encouragement, helping you stay on track and committed to your ketogenic or low carb lifestyle.
- Online Coaching Programs: Consider enrolling in online coaching programs or support groups led by certified coaches or nutrition professionals specializing in ketogenic or low carb nutrition. These programs offer personalized guidance, accountability, and support to help you navigate your dietary journey with confidence and success.

By actively participating in supportive communities and social networks, you can find encouragement, motivation, and practical advice to overcome challenges, celebrate successes, and stay committed to your ketogenic or low carb lifestyle.

Additional Resources and Tools

In addition to the resources mentioned above, there are many other valuable tools and resources available to support your ketogenic or low carb journey. Here are a few additional resources to explore:

- Nutritional Supplements: Consider incorporating nutritional supplements such as vitamins, minerals, and herbal extracts to support your overall health and well-being on a ketogenic or low carb diet. Consult with a healthcare professional or registered dietitian to determine which supplements may be beneficial for your individual needs.
- Cooking Equipment and Gadgets: Invest in high-quality cooking equipment and gadgets to make meal prep and cooking more efficient and enjoyable. Consider purchasing kitchen essentials such as a good quality knife set, blender, food processor, or spiralizer to help you prepare delicious and nutritious meals with ease.
- Educational Books and Podcasts: Explore educational books, podcasts, and audiobooks on topics related to ketogenic or low carb nutrition, health, and wellness. Look for titles by

reputable authors and experts in the field, and choose resources that align with your interests and goals.
- Mindfulness and Stress Management Resources: Incorporate mindfulness and stress management techniques into your daily routine to support your overall well-being on a ketogenic or low carb diet. Explore resources such as meditation apps, relaxation exercises, or stress management books to cultivate resilience and emotional well-being.
- Medical and Professional Support: If you have specific health concerns or dietary restrictions, seek guidance from qualified healthcare professionals or registered dietitians who specialize in ketogenic or low carb nutrition. They can provide personalized recommendations and support to help you optimize your dietary approach and achieve your health goals.

By exploring these additional resources and tools, you can enhance your ketogenic or low carb journey, deepen your understanding of nutrition and wellness, and empower yourself to make informed decisions for your health and well-being.

Practical resources and tools play a vital role in supporting success and adherence to ketogenic and low carb diets. From meal planning apps to educational websites, tracking tools, supportive communities, and additional resources, these tools provide valuable information, guidance, and support to help you navigate your dietary journey with confidence and ease. By incorporating these resources into your routine and staying engaged with supportive communities, you can optimize your ketogenic or low carb lifestyle for long-term health and wellness. Stay tuned for the following chapters, where we'll delve deeper into advanced strategies, practical tips, and additional insights for optimizing your ketogenic or low carb journey.

Unraveling the Cookbook Secrets of Keto and Low Carb Living

EMBRACING THE KETO AND LOW CARB LIFESTYLE FOR HEALTH AND WELLNESS

Throughout this comprehensive guide, we've delved into the intricacies of the ketogenic and low carb diets, exploring their origins, scientific principles, practical applications, and advanced strategies for optimization. From understanding the metabolic mechanisms behind ketosis to navigating common challenges and pitfalls, we've provided a wealth of information and resources to empower you on your journey towards improved health and wellness.

Understanding the Basics: We began by laying the foundation of understanding, explaining the fundamental principles of the ketogenic and low carb diets. By restricting carbohydrate intake and increasing fat consumption, these dietary approaches shift the body's primary fuel source from glucose to ketones, leading to metabolic benefits such as weight loss, improved insulin sensitivity, and enhanced cognitive function.

Exploring Health Benefits: We explored the extensive array of health benefits associated with ketogenic and low carb diets, ranging from weight loss and blood sugar regulation to increased energy levels and mental clarity. By harnessing the body's natural ability to burn fat for fuel, individuals can experience profound improvements in overall health and well-being, with potential therapeutic applications for various chronic conditions and metabolic disorders.

Practical Implementation: We provided practical guidance and tips for implementing ketogenic and low carb diets into your daily life, from meal planning and recipe ideas to grocery shopping tips and dining out strategies. By emphasizing whole, nutrient-dense foods and prioritizing quality fats, proteins, and non-starchy vegetables, individuals can nourish their bodies while enjoying delicious and satisfying meals that support their dietary goals.

Navigating Challenges: We addressed common challenges and pitfalls encountered on ketogenic and low carb diets, such as keto flu symptoms, digestive issues, weight loss plateaus, and social and emotional challenges. By providing practical solutions, troubleshooting tips, and mindset shifts, we empowered readers to overcome obstacles and stay on track towards their health and wellness goals with resilience and determination.

Advanced Strategies: We explored advanced strategies and techniques for optimizing ketogenic and low carb lifestyles, including cyclical ketogenic dieting, targeted ketogenic dieting, intermittent fasting, ketone supplementation, and continuous glucose monitoring. By experimenting with these approaches and personalizing their dietary and lifestyle choices, individuals can unlock greater metabolic flexibility, performance, and overall well-being.

Embracing Balance and Sustainability: Throughout our discussion, we emphasized the importance of finding balance and sustainability in the ketogenic and low carb lifestyle. By embracing flexibility, variety, and mindfulness in food choices, prioritizing holistic health practices, and seeking support from communities and professionals, individuals can cultivate a sustainable approach to health and wellness that nourishes the body, mind, and spirit.

The ketogenic and low carb diets offer a powerful framework for optimizing health, achieving weight loss, and enhancing overall well-being. By understanding the underlying principles, implementing practical strategies, and embracing advanced techniques, individuals can harness the transformative potential of these dietary approaches to create lasting change in their lives.

As you embark on your ketogenic or low carb journey, remember that it is not just about the destination, but also about the journey itself. Embrace the process, celebrate small victories, and stay committed to your goals with patience, perseverance, and self-compassion. Whether you're seeking to lose weight, improve metabolic health, or simply feel your best, the principles and practices outlined in this book can guide you towards a healthier, happier, and more vibrant life.

Above all, remember that health is a journey, not a destination. It's about making sustainable choices that support your well-being and enhance your quality of life over the long term. By integrating the principles of the ketogenic and low carb lifestyle into your daily routine, you can unlock your full potential and thrive in mind, body, and spirit.

Thank you for joining us on this transformative journey towards health and wellness. May you

Unraveling the Cookbook Secrets of Keto and Low Carb Living

continue to embrace the power of ketogenic and low carb living to nourish your body, fuel your mind, and elevate your life to new heights. Here's to your health, happiness, and vitality – today, tomorrow, and for years to come.

Printed in Great Britain
by Amazon